Santiago Box Davó

Training on dying for palliative care professionals

Santiago Box Davó

Training on dying for palliative care professionals

Literature review: To reduce fears and improve attitudes in palliative care professionals.

ScienciaScripts

Imprint
Any brand names and product names mentioned in this book are subject to trademark, brand or patent protection and are trademarks or registered trademarks of their respective holders. The use of brand names, product names, common names, trade names, product descriptions etc. even without a particular marking in this work is in no way to be construed to mean that such names may be regarded as unrestricted in respect of trademark and brand protection legislation and could thus be used by anyone.

Cover image: www.ingimage.com

This book is a translation from the original published under ISBN 978-620-3-03548-3.

Publisher:
Sciencia Scripts
is a trademark of
International Book Market Service Ltd., member of OmniScriptum Publishing Group
17 Meldrum Street, Beau Bassin 71504, Mauritius
Printed at: see last page
ISBN: 978-620-3-30118-2

ACKNOWLEDGMENTS

The global coronavirus pandemic exceeds 2.12 million deaths worldwide. In Spain alone, more than fifty-eight thousand people have died. These are the figures as of today, the first day of February 2021, where health workers and the world continue to struggle.

For this reason, we would like to thank all the healthcare personnel for their work, who have been ignored and mistreated so many times up to this point. To all of them, who have been accompanying and caring for the patients in everything and until the end.

Also to my relatives and the rest of the people who have been watching the time pass without being able to do anything, feeling helpless. And of course, to the pets, who are victims of not understanding what is happening, especially to Fito.

To all of them, who have gone out of their way to comply with the rules and prevent the virus from spreading, thank you!

The Hurricane Train

"I went to the woods because I wanted to live deliberately; to deal

only with the essential facts of life.

and see if I could learn everything she had to teach me. I didn't want to

find out at the hour of death that I hadn't lived."

Henry David Thoreau - I Went into the Woods

INDEX:

ACKNOWLEDGMENTS 1

TABLE OF CONTENTS: 3

SUMMARY: 4

INTRODUCTION: 5

1. Conceptualization of death 5

2. Attitudes toward death 6

3. Pedagogy of death 8

4. Attitudes and training of health professionals 10

MATERIAL AND METHODS: 14

Search strategy 14

Inclusion criteria 15

Exclusion criteria 15

Data extraction 16

RESULTS: 20

TABLE 1: Information on the article and sample used in this study 20

Description of selected items 40

DISCUSSION 42

Limitations of the study 44

BIBLIOGRAPHY 45

SUMMARY:

Introduction: An issue as transcendental as death requires adequate preparation for those who deal directly with it, highlighting from this group the professionals working in palliative care services. This learning will have an effective influence on patients or people who are in situations facing death and their surrounding environment, because the care provided will be of better quality, from a biopsychosocial point of view.

Objective: To review the available literature on the effectiveness of training in palliative care units to reduce the level of anxiety and fear and improve attitudes in nursing professionals.

Methodology: A great variety of studies were obtained from different electronic searches in databases such as: Medline, CINAHL, PsycInfo. Manual searches were also carried out and a reference search was performed. Finally, a total of 16 articles from different countries were included in the study for the investigation and respective analysis of the data obtained. In this analysis, two variables were kept in mind at all times: emotions and attitudes of professionals on the subject of death.

Results: Of the set of selected studies, it should be noted that all showed statistically relevant differences in the attitude and behavior reducing the values of anxiety and fear of death ($p \leq 0.05$), once the training plan on death was carried out in nursing students and professionals in palliative care units.

Conclusion: The activities carried out on death and palliative care show that it is possible to reduce the levels of anxiety and fear of professionals working in palliative care units, in addition to bringing about changes in attitudes and behaviors towards death.

Keywords: palliative care, death, continuing nursing education, anxiety, nursing staff.

INTRODUCTION:

1. Conceptualization of death

The human being's attitude towards death has undergone changes, it has gone through different conceptual stages throughout history, as there have been significant changes in the way of facing it. From the High Middle Ages, where death was contemplated in a more "domestic" way, that is to say, closer, it has slowly evolved towards another way of contemplating death. Nowadays, above all, there is an attempt to achieve a "dignified death" and at the same time to distance it from the family context. Moreover, this event, death, is still an embarrassing moment, a scenario that goes beyond our schemes and, in the same way, is presented as a situation of frustration, which cannot be prevented. [3, 9, 12]

Throughout the evolution of knowledge and thought about death, changes have appeared, the transfer of tombs, niches and crypts from the populations themselves to the outside of the same (started during the time of Napoleon with the aim of improving health and hygiene), the origin of death (including the transition from infectious to chronic/degenerative diseases), the orientation (from spirituality to scientific-technical development), quality of life, legal judgments... [3, 5, 6, 12]

Today's world, despite the progress made on this issue, still gives rise to a tendency to replicate, refuse, and even hide death. [9, 12, 13, 28]

Currently, there are two aspects of death from the perspective of its judgment:

1. <u>Refusal or refuge</u>: This is the best known, since the event of death has been hidden, distorted or camouflaged by its outright denial.

2. <u>Integrating or educational desire or purpose</u>: A small group observes death as a phase of one's life, something that should be present because it is inevitable. The human being is born and is doomed to death, *"the evolution of consciousness is irreversible, but not gratuitous."* - J.L. Coll (1976)

In the same way, the concept of death has evolved over time. In addition, new concepts about death have been defined by different authors, among these new meanings we find: [6, 11]

Physiological death: Refers to the functions of vital organs when they cease and there is no way to reverse it and maintain the organism.

Clinical death: Moment in which brain activity ends, even though it is possible to keep some organs functioning with artificial help. At this moment, it is when the functioning as a body-mind entity is interrupted.

Sociological death: This refers to the stages of the disease and agonizing situations that terminal patients suffer when contemplating death in a solitary manner, i.e., they have no support or support from their closest environment.

Psychological death: After a great battle, or not, it is the moment in which the patient does not oppose death, but ends up accepting it. This moment anticipates physiological death.

2. Attitudes towards death

Death probably represents a great fear for people and this translates into fear and pain that they usually have to face. This influences both the patient and his or her family. Some theories, such as Freudian theories, talk about how people use defense techniques to avoid and counteract the existence of their own mortality and their fears about death, and are totally unconcerned. This protective or defensive behavior is the origin of the distance that individuals create between life and death. [9, 11, 13, 20, 21]

People do not tend to relate to or understand physical death as just another stage of life, but the image they have of death contributes to their attitude toward life. [11, 13, 20]

A good attitude and conception about death will lead to greater peace when this event approaches, as opposed to anxiety and fear, being the two most relevant and frequent emotional responses that appear during the dying process: [21, 24]

1.) <u>Death anxiety</u>: This situation is defined as behavior in which death gives rise to emotional distress.

This is presented as an accumulation of behaviors and emotions that are understood as harmful psychological reactions such as: alarm, intimidation, restlessness, anger, disruption, harm, fear, among other emotions. [21, 24]

) <u>Fear of death</u>: Fear of death, or also known as thantophobia, of Greek origin: "Thanatos" (death) and "Phobia" (fear or terror). Some authors refer that it can be interpreted as a set of elements such as: fear of the process of dying, fear of early death, fear of feeling a waste, dread of the strange, terror of the deceased. [21, 24]

These emotions are observed in patients throughout the course of death because they go through different stages, in which the behavior and attitude of the terminally ill patient undergoes changes with the passage from one stage to another. There are numerous proposals about the stages through which patients evolve until they reach their final moment, but there is no cohesion because they vary among authors. [6, 11]

Depending on which stage the patient is in, there are five patterns or models of death linked to these. In these stages one can see the different attitudes of people depending on the patient's situation: [6, 11]

<u>Pattern one</u>: Terminal phase that begins when the patient accepts death (psychic death) since it is impossible to cure or reverse the situation. At this point, the patient's immediate environment begins to distance itself (sociological death), the brain ceases its activity (clinical death) and, finally, the organism succumbs (physiological death).

<u>Pattern two</u>: Situation where people, despite not having died, begin to flee or move away from the patient to deny the event that cannot be prevented, death (sociological death). This moment continues with psychic death, followed by physiological death.

<u>Pattern three</u>: The patient does not accept death as well as his close

environment. This gives rise to great astonishment and panic at the moment it arrives.

Pattern four: In this stage, the patient does not wish to continue living, i.e., psychic death. This gives rise to a situation of social rejection despite the efforts of those closest to him to help him cling to life.

Pattern five: It deals with the social rejection of the artificial maintenance of the body after death.

The terminal patient may behave differently during the different stages, and the attitude he or she adopts may have a positive or negative influence on the caregivers when caring for the patient in his or her last moments. This circumstance shows how important it is that the behavior of caregivers should be as appropriate and positive as possible in order to offer a better quality of life to dying patients. This results in a reduction of discomfort and pain, including their family and closest friends during the treatment of the terminally ill patient, taking into account their last wishes and needs in order to fulfill them and satisfy them as far as possible. [15, 16]

Adopting this behavior is necessary because, in a large number of cases, patients in this situation often show signs that give rise to a rejection of the surrounding environment. [15, 16]

Among the different authors and bibliography there is a great consensus that behaviors and attitudes towards death are influenced by a numerous set of variables that may include: age, years of experience, gender, ethnicity, education, religious belief, first experience with death (how it was and how it affected), self-knowledge, personality, duration of illness, presence of pain, culture, profession and unit where they work... among others. [11]

3. Pedagogy of death

Some authors, from their perspective, agree that education has a series of deficiencies and shortcomings, like a cheese with holes, that is, an unfinished pedagogy. Education about death" is treated as a forbidden subject, a taboo subject, but which is necessary and essential, therefore it should be implemented in education. Dying is as common as living, but education is only taught to live. Not adapting the teaching to incorporate it, results in not educating to "live". [4]

Teaching about death is a content that would have to be taught in a global way throughout the educational process, and not in an ad hoc manner. This would become a first stage, a first phase, an elementary education for everyone. [15, 16]

Pedagogy about death should start in stages, from the bottom up, since some researchers agree that this taboo subject should start from infancy to adolescence. With this implementation in teaching, one could speak of life as if it were a tree, that is, death would be the roots that are necessary for its development, because the opposite of death is not life, but ignorance. [4]

The second stage would deal with a subsequent formative approach, a point of view directed to those people who deal with or live through death and all that it entails on a daily basis. Within this stage, healthcare professionals are included. [15, 16]

The reasons why "death" is absent during education are as follows: [3]

> 1. Lack of professional education (There is a pedagogical vacuum in this area, possibly due to the fact that education is delegated to other institutions.)

> 2. Customs and traditions in different environments and contexts (family environment, religions...): As mentioned in the introduction, during the course of history, death was treated more closely in the homes of the population, as it was lived more closely.

With the passage of time, society has evolved, shifting towards a more blurred lifestyle, which is less focused on the family and what it concerns, i.e., its environment. These fundamentals need to be reformed through a basic teaching about death. This training should be adapted to the student's profile, i.e., depending on the age of the individuals, the subject should be taught differently from others, because as human beings develop, their perception of death, the concept they have, also evolves. [4]

A basic training should include some general principles to be addressed, which are: Fear of death, grief and types, to develop techniques for confronting and expressing emotions....

All these topics can be treated and carried out with different learning tools such as: researching (how long does a dog... usually live?...?), anticipatory activities (life cycle of living beings (people, plants, animals...), prevention of (events, accidents, diseases), characteristic situations (loneliness, loss, sadness, aging, deterioration...), relevant sites (natural disasters, act of terrorism...), conversations (poster exhibition, round table...), extracurricular resources (car cemetery or scrapyard, cursed or haunted buildings, uninhabited villages...). Applying these themes in a didactic way is relevant and it is very possible that children do not understand personal experiences about death. This process should be carried out in a more direct way through a second way, such as, for example, through the observation of animals or the media. [4]

In teaching, all the people (teachers, principal, parents...) who surround the students... have different responsibilities. [4]

4. Attitudes and training of healthcare professionals

Earlier, a subsequent teaching, a second phase for healthcare professionals, was mentioned. This is essential because normally, they tend to show an evasive behavior towards patients with poor prognosis. This shows a situation of helplessness and guilt in the professionals themselves and is linked to the proximity of death and the inconvenience of showing feelings. This impediment is presented through close contact with the patient and the family of the deceased. In spite of this, the health care professionals are aware of the importance of paying attention, listening and dialoguing, since they believe they need to give and show themselves as a support in that circumstance (empathy) due to the large number of feelings that arise (fear, disgust, anger, injustice, shock, impotence...), but the big problem they present is that they do not know how to carry it out. [8, 9, 12, 13]

These most common emotions that tend to appear in turn influence the behavior of healthcare workers. There are three of them: anxiety, fear and depression in the face of death. It should be noted that, of these three, the last is the least frequent. [7, 8, 11, 12, 13]

The fear and anxiety related to death are topics that have been reported for centuries, despite this, it is still not known how to reduce the levels of these in professionals, highlighting this group to nurses, who are the ones who live longer these experiences. All this can lead to the health professionals suffering from the well-known "burnout syndrome" (chronic stress due to the link with psychosocial stressors due to the relationship with the patients who are in this terminal process), other mental conditions such as depression can interfere negatively in the performance of their competences. [12, 21, 13]

There are a large number of health care professionals who face death at the end of the patient's life, but there are many among them who interact with a slow death over a long period of time. These professionals just mentioned are those who work in "Palliative Care" services, where they are made up of a multitude of specialties (physicians, nurses, psychologists, assistants and social workers). [7, 11, 26]

This aim to improve and develop the training of professionals is the result of the hard emotional practice and the feeling of discomfort and frustration that comes with dealing with diseases that cannot be cured or solved and, therefore, death is unquestionable. Healthcare workers do not suffer and suffer only from death, but from the whole process involved. For example: mental exhaustion and deterioration, suffering, the slow struggle to reach the end. [7, 13, 29]

Undoubtedly, possibly the most difficult situation in the whole process is reporting bad news, death or announcing an impending death. This can lead to difficult challenges or events for caregivers to deal with. Nursing professionals know the conflict that can arise when dealing with people who reject the upcoming events because they are not prepared to deal with them. [3, 12, 30]

This moment of having to announce bad news can give rise to anxiety in relatives and patients, which translates into an unwillingness or refusal to talk about death or to accompany them during this last stage of life. All this can mean that the suffering of a terminally ill patient can be aggravated by the lack of dialogue and attention from professionals. Normally, this responsibility usually falls on the nursing staff to try to provide help, create the warmest possible atmosphere or emotional well-being. This could be achieved since this category of professional is the closest and the one that dedicates the most time to care, but for this they need good training and coping tools. [7, 8, 29]

Because of this, it is essential to achieve a better teaching and preparation of students (nurses, doctors, assistants...) in order to decrease the levels of anxiety related to care in palliative units, it is important to prepare professionals to face death during the development of their work. But this has not only been demanded by the scientific community, but also by the professionals themselves who have requested this training, for example: health care professionals (nurses, doctors, students...), teachers, experts in ethics according to the literature. [21, 26]

The literature in Spain on professionals working and providing care in palliative care units is very heterogeneous. To begin with, one study selected all the information related to nursing careers in universities where palliative care was included in the curriculum. The result of the investigation was that palliative care was present in almost all the faculties, but only in half of them was it compulsory for students. [7, 8, 29]

Secondly, if we compare the same situation, but with medical schools, the results are even more deficient. It is true that, with the passage of time, palliative care has been gradually incorporated into training, but in spite of this, at the present time, not even 50% of the study plans include a subject on palliative care. [21, 26]

After what has been stated in the literature and assessing the situation today, it is not surprising that two of the studies on palliative care pedagogy in Spain deal with the importance and essentiality of training in palliative care for health care professionals, since during the previous two decades they mentioned the insufficiency of training programs. They also believe that it would be necessary to suggest the creation of new specialties such as palliative care within nursing. This is because these professionals would be capable and feel prepared, if they had some skills and communication tools, to remove their emotional reactions from the patients and be able to help them as much as possible in their needs, dedicate time to the perception of their situation or clarify all the doubts or problems they may have. [11, 15, 16, 21]

All the literature consulted comments on training in palliative care as the main argument. They are professionals whose aim is to accompany and comfort the patient during the process of illness and adaptation to the emotions and events they are going through, as they can suffer from high levels of vulnerability.

To be able to control and reduce these levels, point out the importance, again, of expressing feelings and how essential it is for the professional to be able to sit with the patient, look at them and listen to them. This is the work that professionals must do, since they are working with a near but slow death. [6, 15, 16]

The main purpose of this research is to analyze the effectiveness of death education in palliative care to reduce the level of anxiety and fear and to improve attitudes to provide better care to patients.

MATERIAL AND METHODS:

Search strategy

The procedure followed to obtain important documents was through electronic searches in different databases such as MEDLINE (Pubmed), CINAHL and PsycInfo between the years 2000 and 2020, this being the search time interval for this research. The search pattern was set to acquire original studies on interventions about training interventions in palliative care units to reduce the level of anxiety and fear and improve attitudes in nursing professionals.

For the search model, an approach was carried out to obtain original studies and papers dealing with palliative care training in nursing professionals.

The search plan was designed to obtain interesting and original research with the use of several terms in Spanish and English: cuidados paliativos / palliative care, muerte / death, educación en enfermería / education, nursing, continuing, ansiedad / anxiety, personal de enfermería / nursing staff.

The first step was to carry out searches using the descriptors and thesauri of each of the databases that were related to the search terms.

Then, with the idea of increasing the sensitivity of the method, despite increasing the "noise". For this purpose, lists of key terms obtained through the DeCS - MeSH were extensively created, which were linked to the search words in order to obtain all data and documents whose titles and/or abstracts contained these terms.

During the two techniques executed, the descriptors were linked to each other by means of *Boolean* operators: key terms were obtained by using *OR* or OR and, for each defining word or search descriptor, they were linked with the AND or AND operator.

From among the five descriptors chosen as keywords, each term was combined with the rest, but without using all of them at the same time. First, the descriptors "nursing staff" and "palliative care" were linked in the title and abstract (AND), and the rest of the descriptors that could be found in any field (OR) were joined to the first search performed (AND). The results of both searches are shown in the figures below (Figures 1, 2 and 3).

However, despite the results, the data obtained from the electronic searches were refined with manual reviews of the bibliographic references of the selected studies after verifying that they met the inclusion criteria.

The same strategy was used in the two resources used. Attached are two figures of two diagrams that represent how the results were obtained when performing the search (Figure 1, 2 and 3).

Inclusion criteria

The criteria for including the most relevant research were those studies that analyzed the effectiveness of educational interventions such as training in palliative care units to reduce the level of anxiety and improve attitudes in nursing professionals.

The studies that were incorporated were those published within a given time interval, between 2000 and 2020, and which were in Spanish or English.

The research should include sessions (face-to-face or not) with the professionals in order to carry out and put into practice tools and techniques to reduce anxiety and fear levels and to improve their behavior in the face of death and to follow up on it.

In addition, it was also important to observe or verify whether the implementation of training for health professionals led to an improvement or not, and for this reason, only those studies in which follow-up was carried out were taken into account.

Finally, it should be noted that in order to be selected, the research had to be experimental or quasi-experimental.

Exclusion criteria

The studies that were excluded were due to the fact that they were in a language other than English or Spanish.

In the selection of the research studies, the titles and abstracts containing the chosen descriptors were analyzed for their exclusion or inclusion in the review. Of all the studies found that appeared to be important or interesting from the title and abstract for the study, but there were doubts about their inclusion or not, this discrepancy was solved by carrying out a complete reading of the research.

In addition, we discarded those studies in which there was no follow-up after the intervention or training of healthcare workers, since it is not possible to know whether it has been effective over time.

Finally, the last reason for excluding some studies was that during their training process or after completion, they did not explain which method they had used.

Data extraction

Data collection was divided into two parts: information on the study and information on the interventions. The first section deals with information about the methodology carried out, the design selected, the year in which the study was conducted, the place where it was carried out, sociodemographic characteristics (age/gender), and the professionals to whom it was directed.

The second section includes information about the training activities: what the intervention consists of, how long it is carried out, by whom it is developed, the measures that are evaluated as results (in this case two emotions: anxiety and fear), and finally the results obtained.

Finally, the author of this research carried out the data extraction and also used the bibliographic management tool, known as Mendeley, for a better organization of the information and to work in a more orderly and efficient manner.

Figure 1: PubMed search

Búsqueda realizada en la base de datos PUBMED

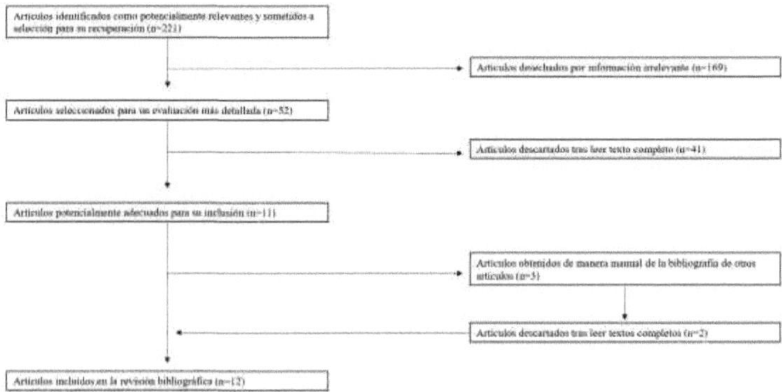

This flowchart shows the data collected through the PubMed database and how research has been selected and excluded according to the criteria set out above.

Figure 2: Search in CINAHL

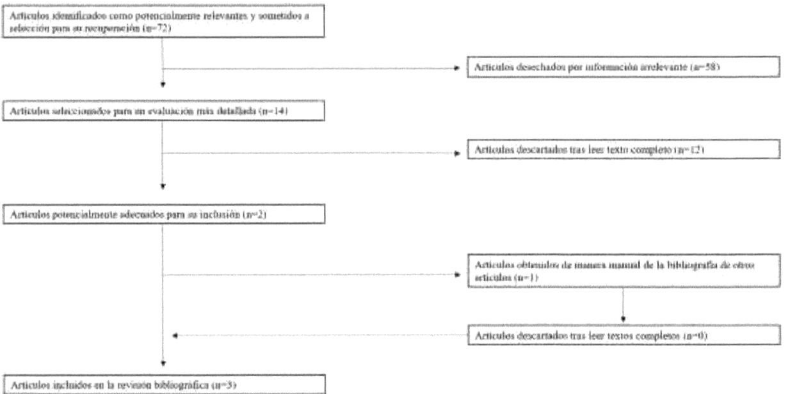

This flowchart shows the data collected through the CINAHL database and how research has been selected and excluded according to the criteria set out above.

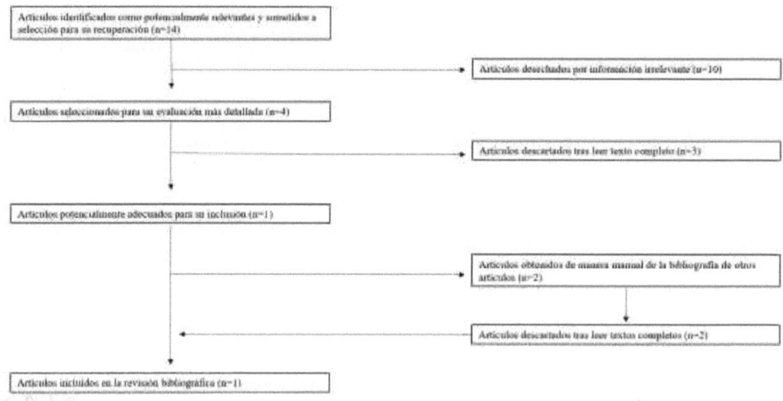

This flowchart shows the data collected through the PsycInfo database and how the investigations have been selected and excluded according to the criteria outlined above.

<h1 style="text-align:center">RESULTS:</h1>

TABLE 1: Information about the article and sample used in this study.

Article	Origin	Design	Sample size		Professional Features
K Hegedeus, et al (2008)	Hungary	Quasi-experimental	toilets	students	Healthcare workers and university nursing students. Predominantly female (although few women). difference) (Mean age= 28.7)
Joaquín Tomás-Sábado and Eulalia Guix Llistuella (2001)	Spain	Quasi-experimental	nurses	auxiliaries	Nurses and assistants. Predominantly female (mean age= 34.84 years).
Cara L.Wallace, et al (2017).	USA	Quasi-experimental			University students enrolled in the subject "Death and Dying". Predominantly female (19-58 years old)

Article	Origin	Design	Sample size	Professional Features
Maritza Maza Cabrera et al (2009)	Spain	Quasi-experimental		Nurse practitioners. Predominantly female (mean age===). 29.87)
Alan E. Steawart (2000)	USA	Quasi-experimental	240	Nurses. Predominantly male (although with a small number of male nurses). difference) (Mean age= 44.2)
Ramón Colell Brunet, et al (2003)	Spain	Quasi-experimental		First-year nursing students. Predominance of gender female. (Average age 19.9)
Mercedes Zavala Gutiérrez, et al. (2008)	Chile	Quasi-experimental		Nurses. Predominantly female. (Average age= 33.67)

Article	Origin	Design	Sample size	Professional Features
Carol Gouveia Melo and Jenny Bilings (2018)	Portugal	Quasi-experimental	22	Nursing professionals, the majority of whom were female. mean = 44.6 years)
Montserrat Edo Gual (2015)	Spain	Quasi-experimental	772	Nursing students. Predominantly female (mean age= 20.54).
Irene Searles McClatchey and Steve King (2015)	USA	Experimental		Nursing. Predominantly female. (Average age = 28.21)
SH Wong (2012)	China	Quasi-experimental		Nursing students. Predominantly female (but with little difference) (Mean age= 19-73). years)

Article	Origin	Design	Sample size		Professional Features
Amor Aradilla Herrero (2006)	Spain	Quasi-experimental			3rd year nursing class enrolled in palliative care. Predominance of female gender (20-25 years old)
And Masuda, et al (2006)	Japan	Quasi-experimental	1004		Nursing students, the majority were female (Mean age= 23.8)
Jane M. Kurz and Evelyn R. Hayes (2006)	USA	Quasi-experimental			Nurses. Predominantly female (Mean age= 43.7).
Esther Mok, et al (2019)	Japan	Quasi experimental			Nursing students. Predominance of female gender. (mean age= 22.3)
Lourdes Chocarro González (2010)	Spain	Experimental	nurses	physicians	Nursing and health care professionals medicine. Majority female nurses (average age 27.2 years).

TABLE 2: Information about the intervention carried out in each of the studies

Study	Action / Intervention	What does it consist of?	Duration	Who carried out?	Measuring instrument	Variable result	Statistical values
K Hegedeus, et al (2008)	Training on death and use of the questionnaire "Fear of death".	Mandatory training for professionals and students. Course taught at the university and hospital. Subject related to the fear of death	Duration: 14 days (2 hours each day) Follow-up: 3 months	Nursing	Death Anxiety Scale (DAS) Attitude Towards Death Questionnaire (CAM)	Attitudes and anxiety in the face of death	Different results in readings between pre- and post-intervention measurements. P ≤0.05

Study	Action / Intervention	What does it consist of?	Duration	Who carried out?	Measuring instrument	Variable result	Statistical values
Joaquín Tomás and Eulalia Guix Llistuell a (2001)	Interventions to support and guide the patient in the process of dying.	Voluntary intensive training, free of charge during working hours. The objective is to identify anxiety and deal with it by strategy.	Duration: 35 hours (4 days) Follow-up: not indicated	Teachers with a specialty in Palliative Care	Death Anxiety Scale (DAS) Attitude Towards Death Questionnaire (CAM)	Anxiety and attitudes towards death	Different results in readings between pre- and post-intervention measurements. P=0.038

Study	Action / Intervention	What does it consist of?	Duration	Who carried out?	Measuring instrument	Variable result	Statistical values
Cara L. Wallace, et al (2017).	Death education and use of a pre- and post-test on attitudes towards death.	Mandatory and classroom training. Treats behaviors before the first experience of death.	Duration: not indicated Follow-up: 6 months	Teachers with a specialty in Palliative Care	Death anxiety inventory (DAI) Attitude Towards Death Questionnaire (CAM)	Death anxiety and attitudes	Different results in readings between pre- and post-intervention measurements. P=0.026

Study	Action / Intervention	What does it consist of?	Duration	Who carried out?	Measuring instrument	Variable result	Statistical values
Maritza Maza Cabrera et al (2009)	To assess the behavior and attitude of nurses in the face of patient death (related to factors that condition it)	Voluntary training conducted in the boardroom. It deals with the most frequent conditioning factors that influence the attitude of the professionals	Not indicated	Nursing teachers with a specialty	3 scales: 1. Biosociodemographic Characteristics (adapted), 2. Death Attitude Measurement Scale, 3. (CAM)	Attitude towards death	Different results in readings between pre- and post-intervention measurements. P= 0.024

Study	Action / Intervention	What does it consist of?	Duration	Who carried out?	Measuring instrument	Variable result	Statistical values
Alan E. Stewart (2000)	Training on the first experience of death before and after the patient's death	Voluntary training. Addresses communication techniques for reporting bad news.	Duration: 24 weeks (4 hours per week) Follow-up: 3 years	Teachers who teach the subject of palliative care	Death Anxiety Scale (DAS) Scale for Measuring Attitude to Death	Death anxiety and death notification experience (attitude)	Different results in readings between pre- and post-intervention measurements. P= 0.042

Study	Action / Intervention	What does it consist of?	Duration	Who carried out?	Measuring instrument	Variable result	Statistical values
Ramón Colell Brunet, et al (2003)	Performance to examine students' behaviors, beliefs, and emotions in the face of death	During the palliative care course. Volunteer.	Duration: 6 hours per week Follow-up: 4 months	Teachers who teach the subject of palliative care	Scale of professional preferences The death anxiety scale, death anxiety scale and questionnaire of factors that help to die	Students' preferences, anxiety and attitudes towards death	Different results in readings between pre- and post-intervention measurements. P=0.026

Study	Action / Intervention	What does it consist of?	Duration	Who carried out?	Measuring instrument	Variable result	Statistical values
Mercedes Zavala Gutiérrez, et al (2008)	Use of questionnaires to assess nursing attitudes	Voluntary training, related to the attitudes of professionals during the death of a patient.	Duration and follow-up: not indicated	Nursing teachers	Attitude to Death Measurement Scale and the Attitude to Death Questionnaire (CAM).	Attitude and death	Different results in readings between pre- and post-intervention measurements. P= 0.0014

Study	Action / Intervention	What does it consist of?	Duration	Who carried out?	Measuring instrument	Variable result	Statistical values
Carol Gouveia Melo and Jenny Bilings (2018).	Questionnaires and actions (AMARA) about anxiety and fear of death	Group therapies and voluntary experimental interventions, treating simulated cases	Duration: 36 hours (6 days) Follow-up: not indicated	Palliative care educators	Fear Evaluation Scale (FES)	Anxiety and fear of death	Different results in readings between pre- and post-intervention measurements. P=0.007

Study	Action / Intervention	What does it consist of?	Duration	Who carried out?	Measuring instrument	Variable result	Statistical values
Montserrat Edo Gual (2015)	End-of-life training program to reduce levels of anxiety and fear of death	Mandatory training to reduce anxiety levels through class attendance of students.	Duration: not stated Follow-up: not indicated	Nursing teachers	Collet-Lester Fear of Death Scale-CLFDS and Death Anxiety Inventory	Anxiety and fear of death	Different results in readings between pre- and post-intervention measurements. P= 0.038

Study	Action / Intervention	What does it consist of?	Duration	Who carried out?	Measuring instrument	Variable result	Statistical values
Irene Searles McClatchey and Steve King (2015).	Training classes on fear and anxiety in the face of death	Voluntary training given during the trimester. Palliative care topics	Duration: 16 weeks Follow-up: not indicated	Nursing teachers	Death anxiety inventory [DAI] Collet-Lester Fear of Death Scale-CLFDS	Anxiety and fear of death	Different results in readings between pre- and post-intervention measurements. P= 0.021

Study	Action / Intervention	What does it consist of?	Duration	Who carried out?	Measuring instrument	Variable result	Statistical values
Amor Aradilla Herrero and Joaquín Tomás Sábado (2006)	Educational performance on emotions about death.	On-site training oriented to the recognition of one's own and other people's emotions	Duration: 30 hours Follow-up: not indicated	Nursing faculty	Death anxiety inventory (DAI)	Death anxiety	Different results in readings between pre- and post-intervention measurements. P = 0.023

Study	Action / Intervention	What does it consist of?	Duration	Who carried out?	Measuring instrument	Variable result	Statistical values
SHW ong (2012)	Intervention to understand the link between beliefs and death itself.	Voluntary assignment about unpaid palliative care in the faculty.	Duration: 9 weeks (3,5h/week) 8 months (follow-up)	Nursing faculty	Superstition Paranormal Scale Belief	Beliefs and anxiety about death	Different results in readings between pre- and post-intervention measurements. P=0.03

Study	Action / Intervention	What does it consist of?	Duration	Who carried out?	Measuring instrument	Variable result	Statistical values
Y Masuda, et al (2006)	Death training aimed at reducing anxiety levels	Elective and voluntary death training provided at the university.	Duration: not indicated Follow-up: 2 years	Nursing faculty	Death anxiety inventory [DAI]	Death anxiety	Different results in readings between pre- and post-intervention measurements. P=0.041

Study	Action / Intervention	What does it consist of?	Duration	Who carried out?	Measuring instrument	Variable result	Statistical values
Jane M. Kurz and Evelyn R. Hayes (2006)	Course on Anxiety (ELNEC) at nurses in the face of death	ELNEC course oriented to the problem-based technique linked to the anxiety of healthcare workers	Duration: not indicated Follow-up: 6 months	Palliative care teachers	Death anxiety inventory [DAI]	Death anxiety	Different results in readings between pre- and post-intervention measurements. $P \leq 0.05$

Study	Action / Intervention	What does it consist of?	Duration	Who carried out?	Measuring instrument	Variable result	Statistical values
Esther Mok, et al (2001)	Problem-based training to reduce death anxiety levels	Training delivered with problem-based tools at university level	Duration: 3 months (3h/week) Follow-up: 1 year	Teachers with a specialty	Death anxiety inventory [DAI]	Death anxiety	Different results in readings between pre- and post-intervention measurements. P= 0.032

Study	Action / Intervention	What does it consist of?	Duration	Who carried out?	Measuring instrument	Variable result	Statistical values
Lourdes Chocarro González (2010)	Death education to reduce anxiety	Intensive voluntary training in the palliative care unit boardroom to discuss strategies for communication.	Duration: 15 hours Follow-up: not indicated	Health teachers	Death anxiety inventory [DAI]	Death anxiety	Different results between pre- and post-intervention measurements. P= 0.038

Description of selected items

The description of the data obtained from the articles will be divided into two parts, in the same way as found in the tables.The results in Table 1 show a large number of articles from different origins, i.e., different cultures, but with a predominance of studies in Spain followed by those from the United States. The designs of the studies were "Quasi-experimental" except for a couple that were experimental. [1, 2, 5, 7, 11, 13-16, 21, 24-27, 29, 30] The research samples ranged from 39 to 1004 participants, resulting in a large difference in sample sizes between the research studies. Among the studies, the individuals had different characteristics including professionals from different specialties (doctors, nurses and assistants) and students. The presence of students caused the mean age ranges to be very disparate between students and professionals across studies. This meant that the mean age range was very different, with students ranging from 19.9 to 23.8 years, and professionals from 27.2 to 44.6 years, according to the study. The female gender was more predominant in almost all the researches, but not in all of them, this is due to the fact that nowadays the professions dedicated to the care of people are usually still dominated by women, although with the passage of time a tendency to balance in the teams is being seen. [1, 2, 5, 7, 11, 13-16, 21, 24-27, 29, 30]

It is important to point out that in the studies where the training is carried out in a face-to-face and obligatory manner with all the members of the unit, more positive results were obtained, due to the fact that the follow-up is easier compared to the rest of the interventions. [5, 13, 15, 26, 30]

The results in Table 2 were interpreted in two parts, firstly, the actions aimed at dealing with the attitudes and behaviors towards death of health care workers and, on the other hand, the investigations focused on the anxiety that death itself caused.

In the first place, the investigations oriented to behaviors or attitudes were a total of seven. In the rest, most of them, formative classes on the attitude about death were conducted, but treating the topic to be worked on in a different way.

These interventions were face-to-face and most of them were voluntary. The training was carried out in different places such as: the university (Palliative Care course, assembly hall...) or the hospital (meeting room, Palliative Care services...). [1, 2, 5, 7, 11, 13, 14]

The topics covered in the different interventions were the following: attitudes towards the first experience of death (fear, avoidance...), some of the factors that affected and conditioned the participants according to (ethnicity, gender, religion, age, etc.), factors that condition the way of accepting death (age, gender, ethnicity, ...), influence of beliefs and emotions on attitudes (religion, culture...). Some of the articles were not transparent about the contents they dealt with, they simply stated that they taught "death-related subjects" which included: meaning of death, mourning, fear of the afterlife... [1, 2, 5, 7, 11, 13, 14... 1, 2, 5, 7, 11, 13, 14]

With respect to the time dedicated to interventions in the studies, two things must be differentiated: time dedicated to training and follow-up. Firstly, within the time devoted to training there is an important variety, since the interval ranges from 35 hours, being the shortest, to 96 hours. Secondly, related to follow-up, it ranges from 24 weeks to 3 years depending on the research. This was relevant, the time dedicated to training and follow-up. However, it should be noted that in several studies the duration of the sessions was not indicated, since one did not estimate a specific time,[2,7,11]

The training was carried out by health care professionals, mainly teachers and nursing professionals with a specialty in palliative care. The instruments and methods used to measure the information were: the Attitude to Death Questionnaire (CAM), the Attitude to Death Measurement Scale and the Professional Preferences Scale. [1, 2, 5, 7, 11, 13, 14]

In terms of the effectiveness of the interventions all stood out for showing statistically significant differences in the outcome variables ($p \leq 0.05$). [1, 2, 5, 7, 11, 13, 14]

In second place, the investigations oriented to emotions were nine of the total. A large part of them carried out training about the emotions that appear when death arrives, highlighting anxiety and fear, but it is worth noting that each programming used a different strategy to address the topic to be dealt with, for example: problem-solving (pedagogical classes to learn and solve events that may occur in reality), therapies and group scenarios (presentations of their experiences and carrying out simulations to see what could be improved), recognition and analysis of emotions (individual activity in which the emotions presented by a patient were analyzed)... [15-16, 21, 24-27, 29, 30] All research was carried out on a face-to-face, voluntary and unpaid basis. The courses were held at the universities (classrooms, faculty assembly hall...) as well as at the hospital (palliative care unit). [15-16, 21, 24-27, 29, 30] In the same way as behavioral research, with respect to the duration of the studies, a distinction is made between the time devoted to the preparation and development of the individuals and the time devoted to follow-up and control. With regard to the period devoted to training, there is a variety ranging from 15 to 36 hours. The fact that in this grouping of studies there is not so much disparity may be due to the fact that in many studies these values are not specified. In relation to the duration of controls or follow-up, it varies from 6 months to a maximum of 2 years. [15, 26, 27, 30] With regard to those responsible for providing training in the different studies, the predominance of nursing teachers was noted, although in some studies they were health professionals. Among the measurement instruments chosen, the most predominant was the "Death anxiety inventory (DAI)", but there were also others such as: Superstition Paranormal Paranormal Scale Belief, Collet-Lester Fear of Death Scale-CLFDS, Multidimensional Fear of Death Scale (MFODS) and Fear Evaluation Scale (FES). [15-16, 21, 24-27, 29, 30] Finally, regarding the effectiveness of the studies, all of them showed statistically significant differences in the outcome variable ($p \leq 0.05$) between the experimental and control groups and also in the pre- and post-test groups. [15-16, 21, 24-27, 29, 30]

DISCUSSION

The aim of this review article was to analyze the beneficial effect of training in palliative care units to reduce the level of anxiety and fear and improve attitudes in nursing professionals. In spite of the large amount of research in the literature, and The variety among them was such that only those that carried out a follow-up were chosen.

The study is made up of sixteen articles, of which the majority concluded that the professionals who participated in the training provided managed to improve and decrease their levels of anxiety and fear of death.

Something relevant to point out about the chosen research is that a great variety of techniques and modes can be contemplated as a strategy employed on the number of sessions, duration and follow-up period. Due to this lack of homogeneity, it is difficult to reach a consensus on the most appropriate number, duration and interval of sessions. This complicates the monitoring of the data obtained in a more correct way.

However, despite the above, many studies and researchers reach the consensus that this training should not be a one-time process, as these programs should be repeated in order not to lose the positive effects and what has been learned. For this reason, they recommend a minimum duration of 6 months to observe and compare the effects on professionals, which is not proven.

The training is carried out by qualified health care professionals due to the subject they deal with. It is true that death affects the entire population, but not all people are prepared to deal with this subject.

One group of studies suggests that this training should be included from the earliest stages of life, i.e., infancy. In order to be able to continue such training in a more professional way with the people who will deal with it on a daily basis. [10,19,23]

Teaching about death gives rise to a large number of new concepts and learning that favor giving an answer or solution to all those situations that a person may face. Therefore, educating

The teaching about death favors an education in values and for peace, in short, it teaches you how to live. [7, 19, 22]

Continuing with our argument, training in palliative care has many benefits. Some of the most outstanding ones could be: improvement of communication with the terminal patient and his or her environment, development of empathy, help in decision making... and all these aspects will contribute to achieve a positive attitude in the professionals. [14, 17, 28]

Finally, studies emphasize that life expectancy has increased due to medical advances, but it is essential that healthcare professionals are well trained to work more satisfactorily with patients. [8, 11 22]

Above all, at the moment when medicine can no longer give anything to cure, since there is only the option of caring for the sick until their last moment. Because of this and all that has already been mentioned, healthcare professionals must maintain a positive attitude and behavior when facing this situation. [15, 16, 23]

Limitations of the study

Although the data obtained are convincing, it is important to keep in mind the limitations that have been encountered during this research. The first limitation was the inability to access some published articles. The second is inherent to the use of electronic searches and document retrieval. Sensitivity has always been a priority throughout the strategic process; therefore, electronic database searches were supplemented with manual searches and reference trails. The third, and lastly, was not having considered the use of gray medical literature.

In conclusion, it can be said that training and educational courses on death and palliative care in both university and hospital settings, through follow-up, decrease the levels of anxiety and fear of health care workers and students, modifying their behaviors and attitudes about death by obtaining tools and coping techniques.

BIBLIOGRAPHY

1. Almeida, L. F. de, & Falcão, E. B. M. (2013). *Social representation of death among health professionals: A psychosociological approach from discourse analysis. Psicologia Escolar e Educacional* (Vol. 37). https://doi.org/10.1590/1809-584420143. https://doi.org/10.1590/1809-584420143.

2. Tomás Sábado, J., & Guix Llistuella, E. (2001). Death anxiety: effects of a training course in nurses and nursing assistants. *Enfermería Clínica, 11*(3), 104-109. https://doi.org/10.1016/S1130- 8621(01)73697-2

3. Una, I. A., & La, P. D. E. (2007). EDUCATION FOR LIFE-DEATH:, *17*. Retrieved from https://dialnet.unirioja.es/descarga/articulo/2392479.pdf

4. De, A., & Cortina, M. (2008). La Educación Para La Muerte Como Ámbito Formativo : Más, *5*, 409-424. Retrieved from 15442

5. Wallace, C. L., Cohen, H. L., & Jenkins, D. A. (2017). Transforming students' attitudes and anxieties toward death and loss: the role of earlier death experiences.

6. Pires, J. H. (n.d.). Education for death.

7. Cabrera, M., Zavala Gutiérrez, M., & Merino Escobar, J. M. (2008). Attitude of the nursing professional to the death of patients. *CIENCIA Y ENfERMERIA XV*, (1), 39-48. https://doi.org/10.4067/S0717- 95532009000100006

8. López Palomo, I., & García Sánchez, R. (2008). A nurse's attitude towards death. *Enfermería Docente, 88*, 28-30. Retrieved from les/revistas/ED-88-08.pdf

9. Celma Perdigon, A. G., & Strasser, G. (2015). The dying process and nursing: a relational approach. Theoretical reflections around care in the face of death. *Revista de Saúde Coltiva, 25*(2), 487-500. https://doi.org/10.1590/S0103-73312015000200009

10. Criado-Álvarez, J. J., González González, J., Romo Barrientos, C., Ubeda-Bañon, I., Saiz-Sanchez, D., Flores-Cuadrado, A., ... Mohedano-Moriano, A. (2017). Learning from human cadaveric prosections: Examining anxiety in speech therapy students. *Anatomical Sciences Education, 10*(5), 487- 494. https://doi.org/10.1002/ase.1699

11. Almeida, L. F. de, & Falcão, E. B. M. (2013). *Social representation of death among health professionals: A psychosociological approach from discourse analysis. Psicologia Escolar e Educacional* (Vol. 37). https://doi.org/10.1590/1809-584420143. https://doi.org/10.1590/1809-584420143.

12. Santos, M. A., & Hormanez, M. (2013). The attitude among nursing professionals and students when facing death: a review of the scientific literature of the last decade. *Science & Collective Health, 18*, 2757-2768. https://doi.org/10.1590/S1413-81232013000900031

13. Colell Brunet, R., Limonero García, J. T. . , & Otero, M. D. (2003). Attitudes and emotions in nursing students in the face of death and terminal illness. *Investigación En Salud, V*(2). Retrieved from http://www.redalyc.org/html/142/14250205/%0Ahttp://www.redalyc.org/articulo.oa?id=14250205%0Ahttp://www.redalyc.org/html/142/14250205/%0Ahttp://www.redalyc.org/articulo.oa?id=14250205

14. Melo, C. G., & Billings, J. (2017). Including personal development in palliative care education to address death anxiety. *International Journal of Palliative Nursing, 23*(1), 36-45. https://doi.org/10.12968/ijpn.2017.23.1.36

15. Maza Cabrera, M., Zavala Gutiérrez, M., & Escobar, J. M. (2009). Attitude of the nursing professional to the death of patients. *Ciencia Y Enfermería, 15*(1). https://doi.org/10.4067/S0717-95532009000100006

16. Edo-Gual, M. (2015). Attitudes towards death and related factors of nursing students in the autonomous community of Catalonia. *Doctoral Thesis Actitudes Ante La Muerte Y Factores Relacionados de Los Estudiantes de Enfermería.* , 158. Retrieved from http://www.tdx.cat/handle/10803/317380

17. Onyechi, K. C. N., Onuigbo, L. N., Eseadi, C., Ikechukwu-Ilomuanya, A. B., Nwaubani, O. O., Umoke, P. C. I., ... Utoh-Ofong, A. N. (2016). Effects of rational-emotive hospice care therapy on problematic assumptions, death anxiety, and psychological distress. *International Journal of Environmental Research and Public Health, 13*(9), 1-14. https://doi.org/10.3390/ijerph13090929

18. Brown, A. J., Shen, M. J., Urbauer, D., Taylor, J., Parker, P. A., Carmack, C., ... Bodurka, D. C. (2016). Room for improvement: An examination of advance care planning documentation among gynecologic oncology patients. *Gynecologic Oncology, 142*(3), 525-530. https://doi.org/10.1016/j.ygyno.2016.07.010

19. Collazo, I. V. M., & Tatum, W. O. (2016). Sudden unexpected death in oncology (SUDEP): Are all your patients informed? *Neurologist, 21*(4), 66- 71. https://doi.org/10.1097/NRL.0000000000000083

20. Kim, B. R., Cho, O. H., & Yoo, Y. S. (2016). The effects of Dying Well Education Program on Korean women with breast cancer. *Applied Nursing Research, 30*, 61-66. https://doi.org/10.1016/j.apnr.2015.11.007

21. McClatchey, I. S., & King, S. (2015). The impact of death education on fear of death and death anxiety among human services students. *Omega (United States), 71*(4), 343-361. https://doi.org/10.1177/0030222815572606

22. Cox, C. R., Eaton, S., Ekas, N. V., & Van Enkevort, E. A. (2015). Death concerns and psychological well-being in mothers of children with autism spectrum disorder. *Research in Developmental Disabilities, 45-46*, 229- 238. https://doi.org/10.1016/j.ridd.2015.07.029

23. Stella, M. (2016). Befriending death: A mindfulness-based approach to cultivating self-awareness in counselling students. *Death Studies, 40*(1), 32-39. https://doi.org/10.1080/07481187.2015.1056566

24. Wong, S. H. (2013). Does superstition help ? a study of the role of superstitions and death beliefs on death anxiety, *65*(1), 55-70. Retrieved from http://journals.sagepub.com/doi/pdf/10.2190/OM.65.1.d

25. Hegedus, K., Zana, Á., & Szabó, G. (2008). Effect of end of life education on medical students' and health care workers' death attitude. *Palliative Medicine, 22*(3), 264-269. https://doi.org/10.1177/0269216307086520

26. McClatchey, I. S., & King, S. (2015). The impact of death education on fear of death and death anxiety among human services students. *Omega (United States), 71*(4), 343-361. https://doi.org/10.1177/0030222815572606

27. Kurz, J. M., & Hayes, E. R. (2006). End of life issues action: impact of education. *International Journal of Nursing Education Scholarship, 3*(1), Article 18. https://doi.org/10.2202/1548-923X.1189

28. Mooney, D. C. (2005). Tactical reframing to reduce death anxiety in undergraduate nursing students. *American Journal of Hospice and*

Palliative Medicine, 22(6), 427-432.
https://doi.org/10.1177/1049909105022200607

29. Mok, E., Wai, & Kam-yuet, F. (2002). The issue of death and dying: Employing problem-based learning in nursing education. *Nurse Education Today*, 22(4), 319-329. https://doi.org/10.1054/nedt.2001.0708

30. Stewart, A. E., Lord, J. H., & Mercer, D. L. (2000). A survey of professionals' training and experiences in delivering death notifications. *Death Studies*, 24(7), 611-631. https://doi.org/10.1080/07481180050132811

31. MARTI-GARCIA, Celia, et al. Palliative care training and effect on emotional assessment of death imagery. Palliative Medicine, 2016, vol. 23, no 2, p. 72-78.

32. GALIANA, Laura, et al. Confirmatory validation of the Coping with Death Scale in palliative care professionals. Palliative Medicine, 2017, vol. 24, no 3, p. 126-135.

33. HERNÁNDEZ QUINTERO, Odalys Tomaida, et al. Level of information on palliative care in resident physicians. Educación Médica Superior, 2015, vol. 29, no 1, p. 14-27.

34. GONZÁLEZ, María Cristina. Palliative Care. Towards a medicine of compassion. Salus, 2005, vol. 9, no 1, p. 47-60.

35. ASTUDILLO, W.; MENDINUETA, C.; CASADO, A. How to cope better with losses in palliative care. Revista de la Sociedad Española del Dolor, 2007, vol. 14, no 7, p. 511-526.

36. BOUZA, E. Tizón; TORRADO, R. Vázquez. Nursing in palliative care: hospitalization during the last days of life. Enfermería global, 2004, vol.

3, no 2.

37. PIEDRAFITA-SUSÍN, A. B., et al. Nurses' perceptions, experiences, and knowledge of palliative care. 2015, vol. 26, no 4, p. 153-165.

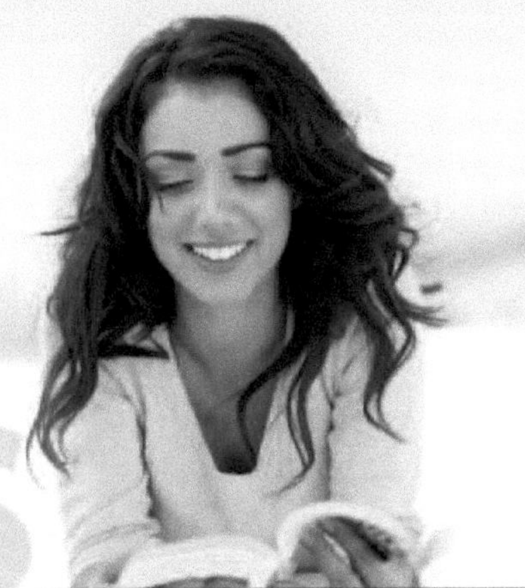

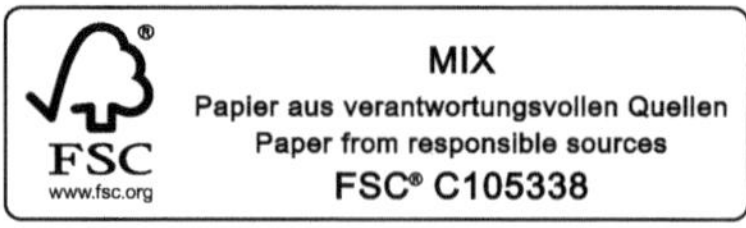

Printed by Books on Demand GmbH, Norderstedt / Germany